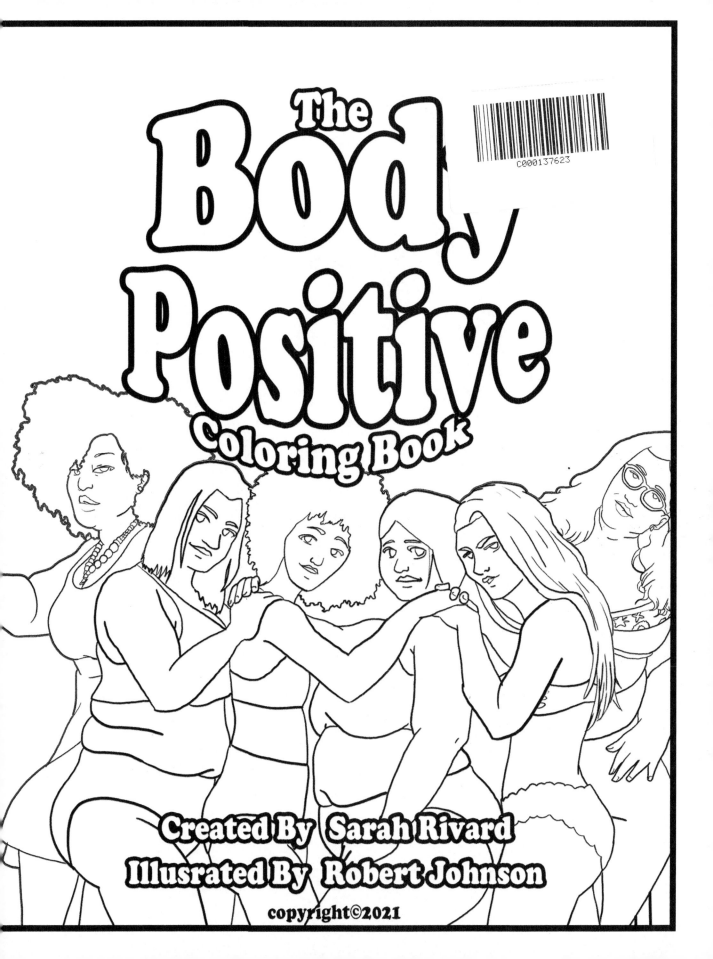

Be Yourself

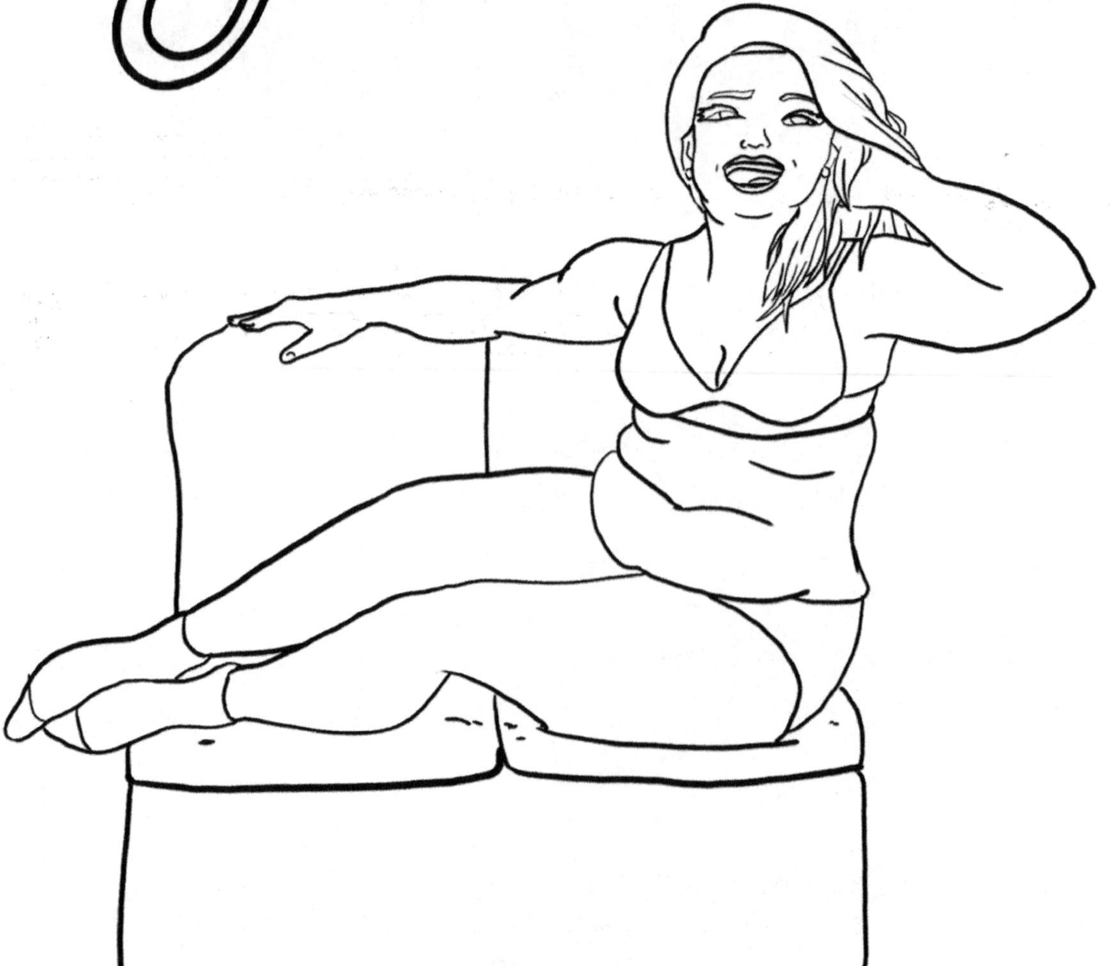

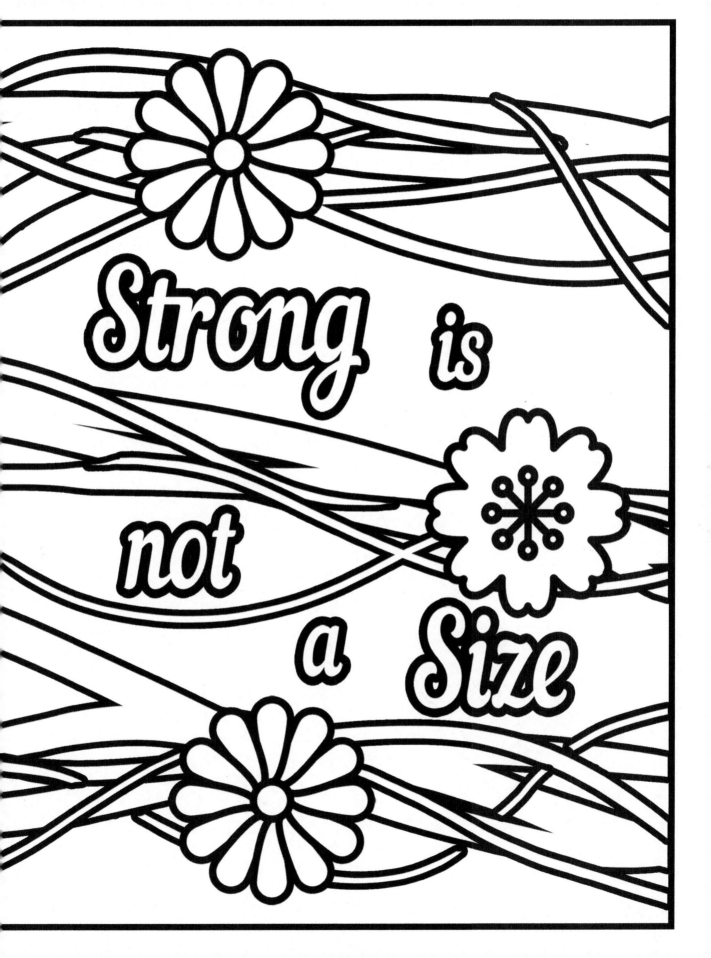

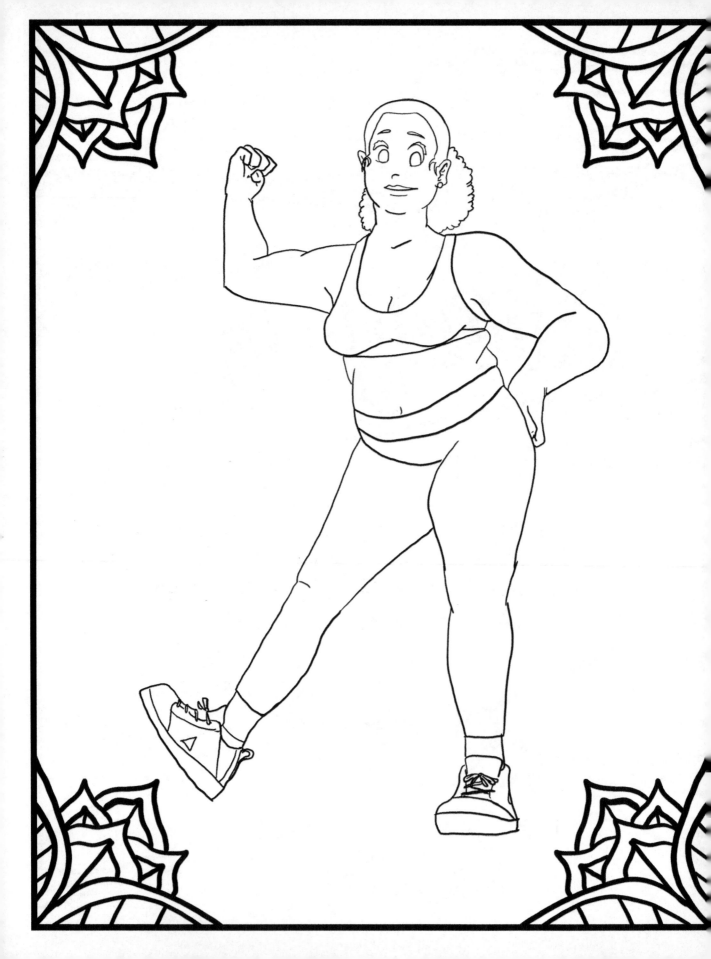

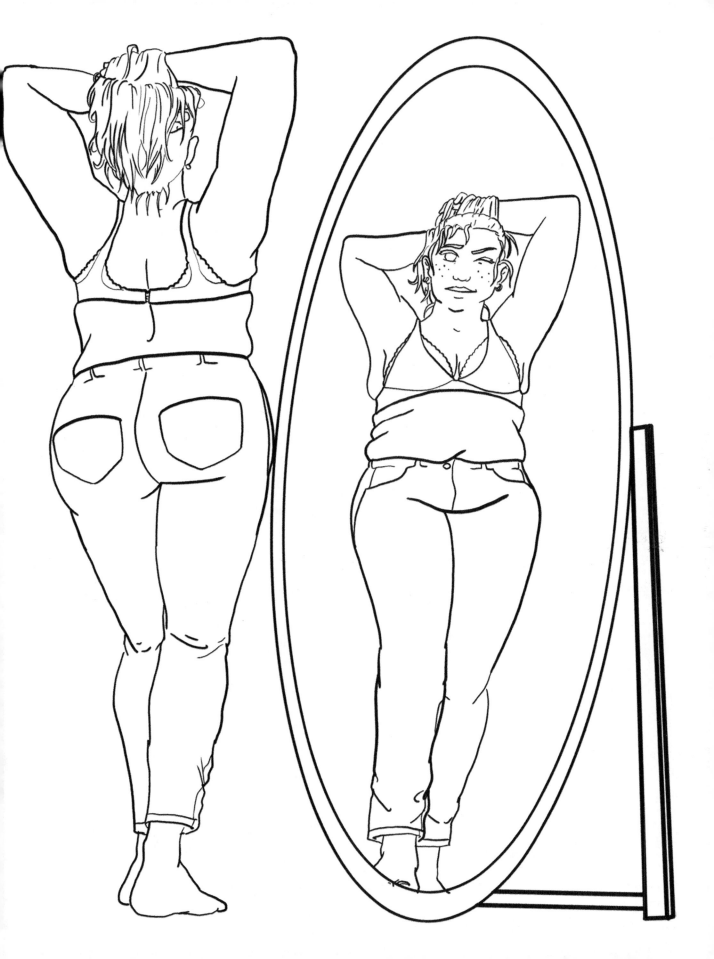

How do you get a

BIKINI

BODY?

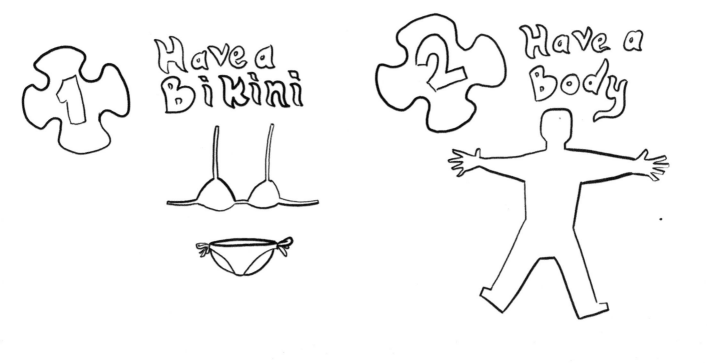

1 Have a Bikini

2 Have a Body

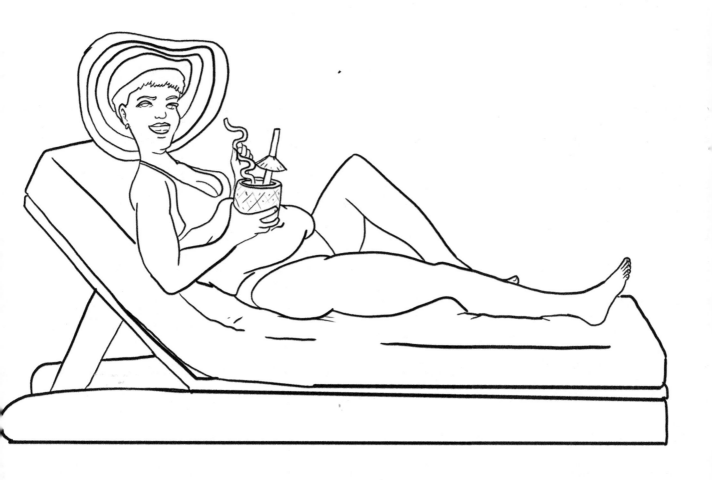

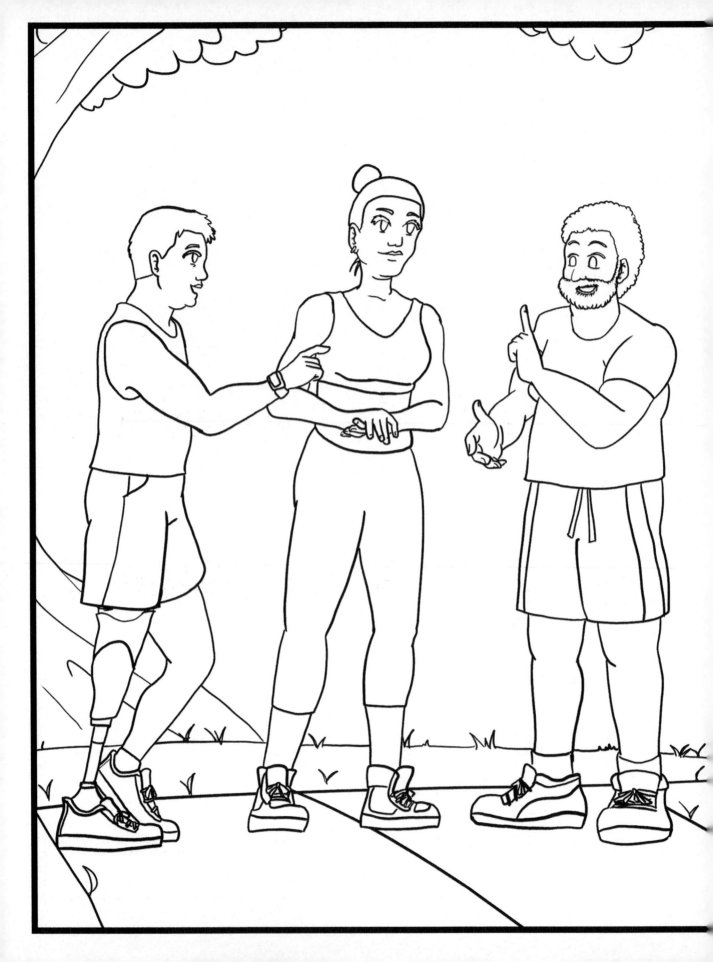

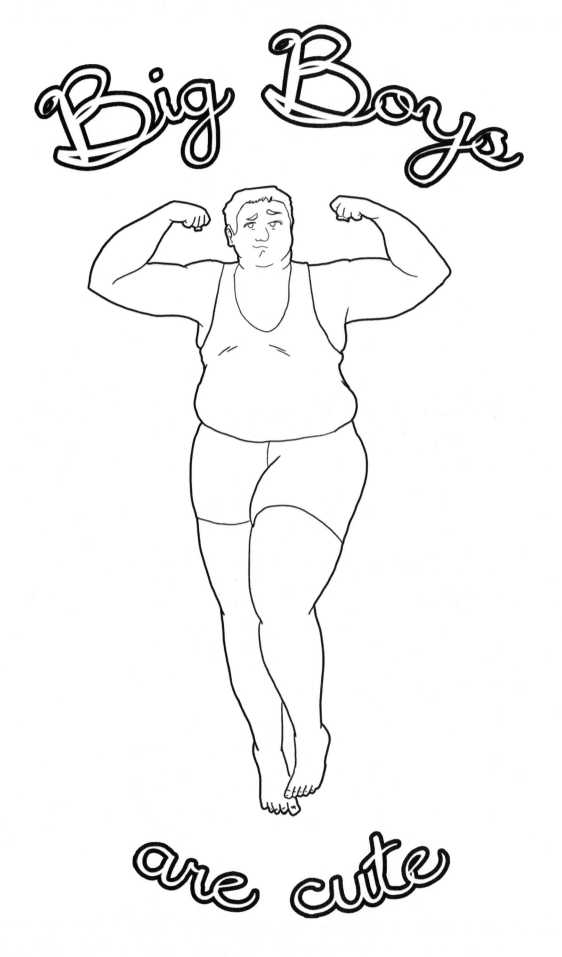

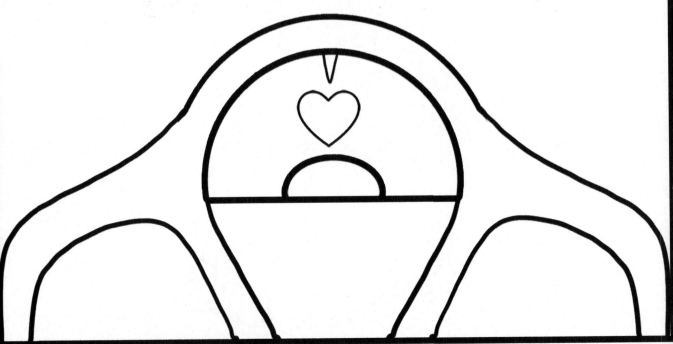

ALL BODIES ARE GOOD BODIES

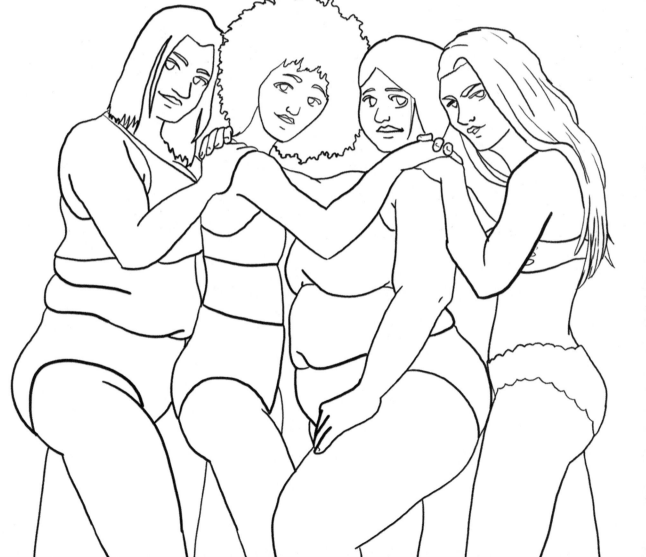

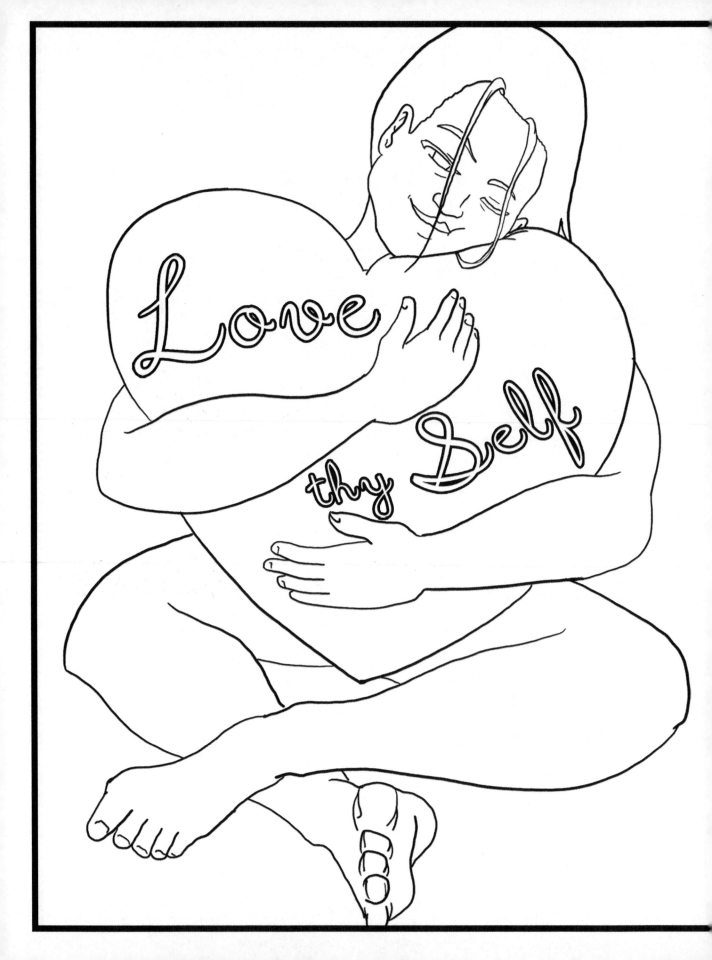

30 Day Body Love Challenge

1. _____
2. _____
3. _____
4. _____
5. _____
6. _____
7. _____
8. _____
9. _____
10. _____
11. _____
12. _____
13. _____
14. _____
15. _____

16. _____
17. _____
18. _____
19. _____
20. _____
21. _____
22. _____
23. _____
24. _____
25. _____
26. _____
27. _____
28. _____
29. _____
30. _____

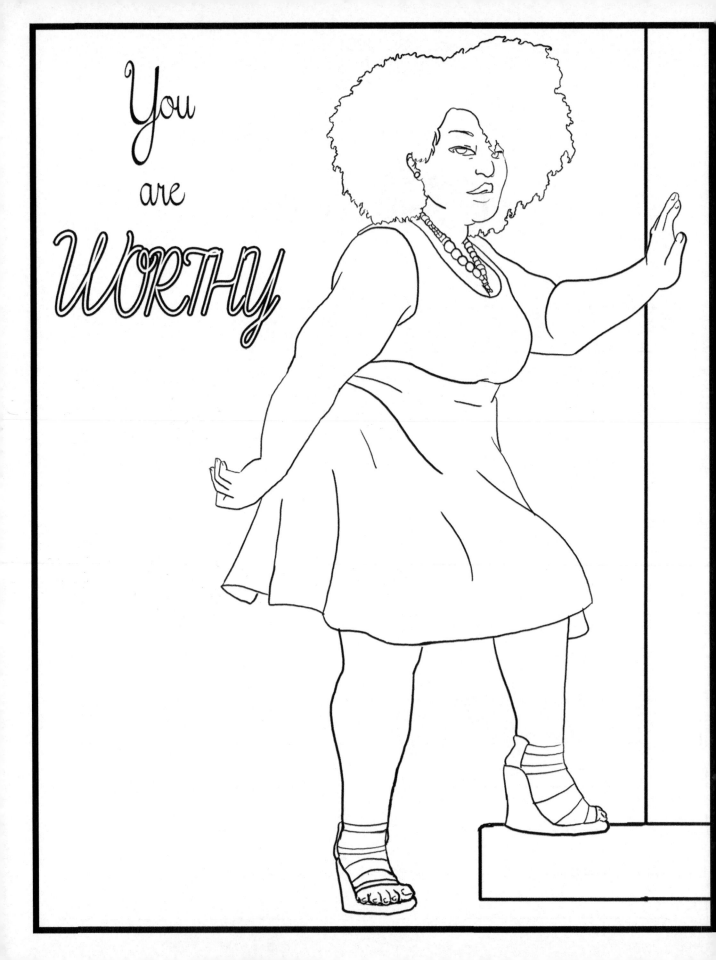

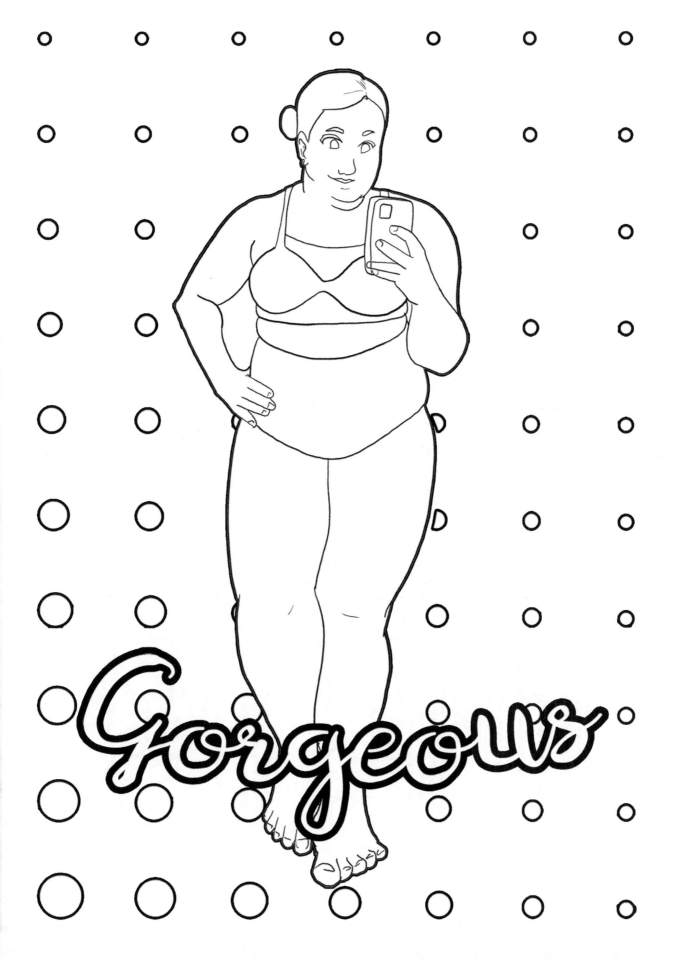

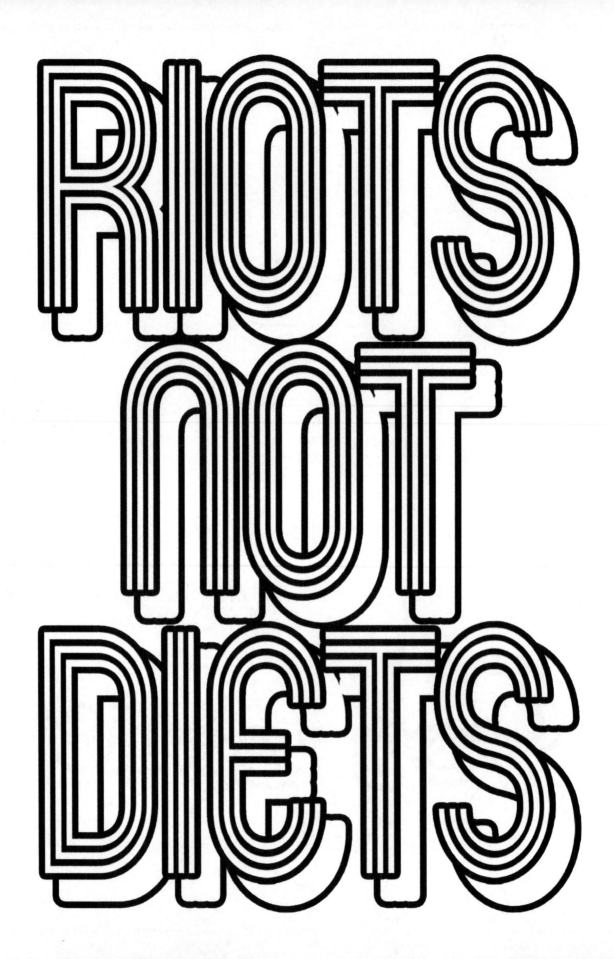

Born
Real
Not
Perfect

Perfect
Not
Real
Born

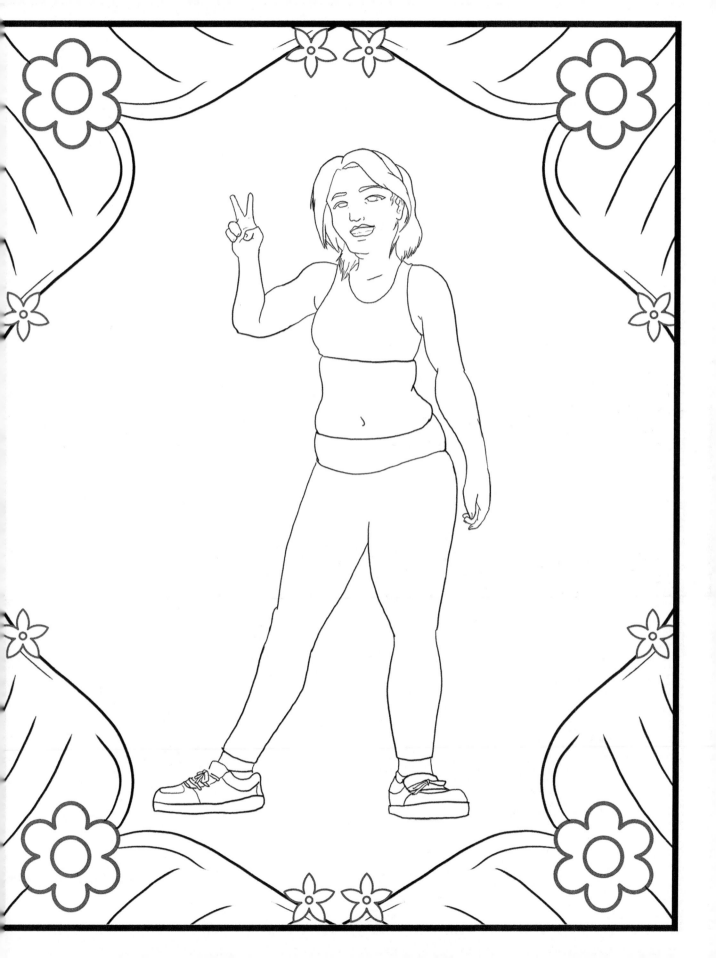

It's okay if all you did today was breathe

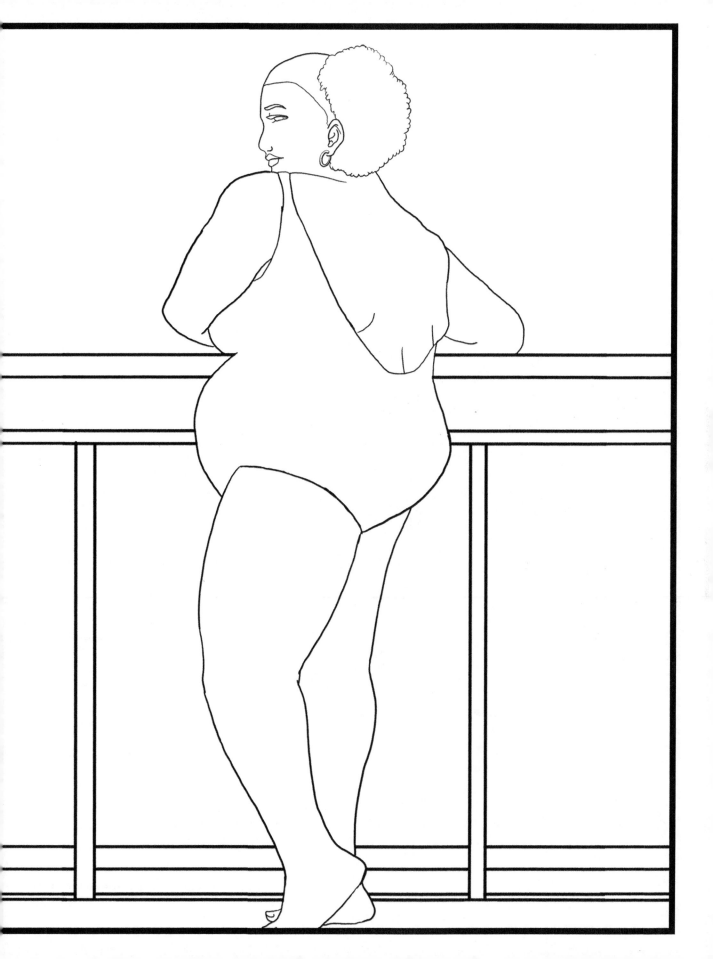

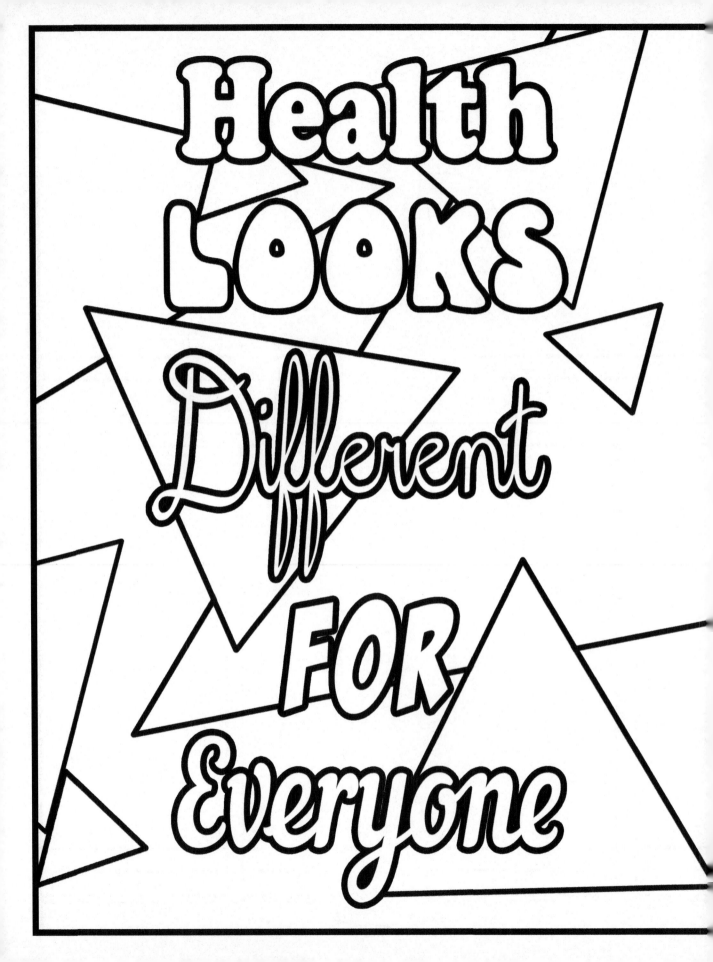

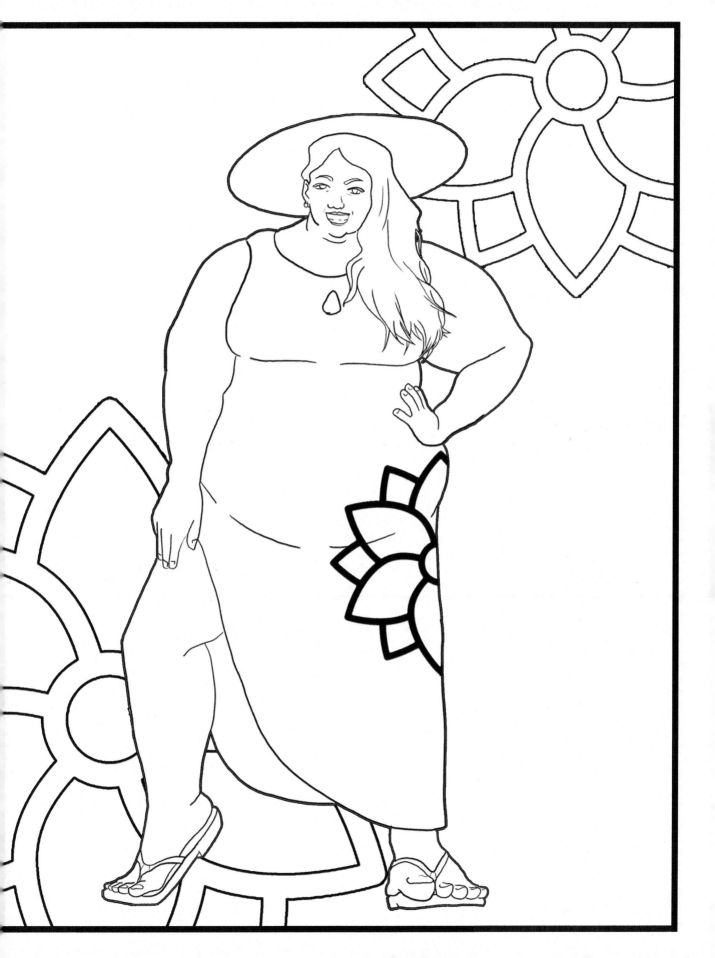

You may be wrestling with your body but...

YOU STILL HAVE TO EAT

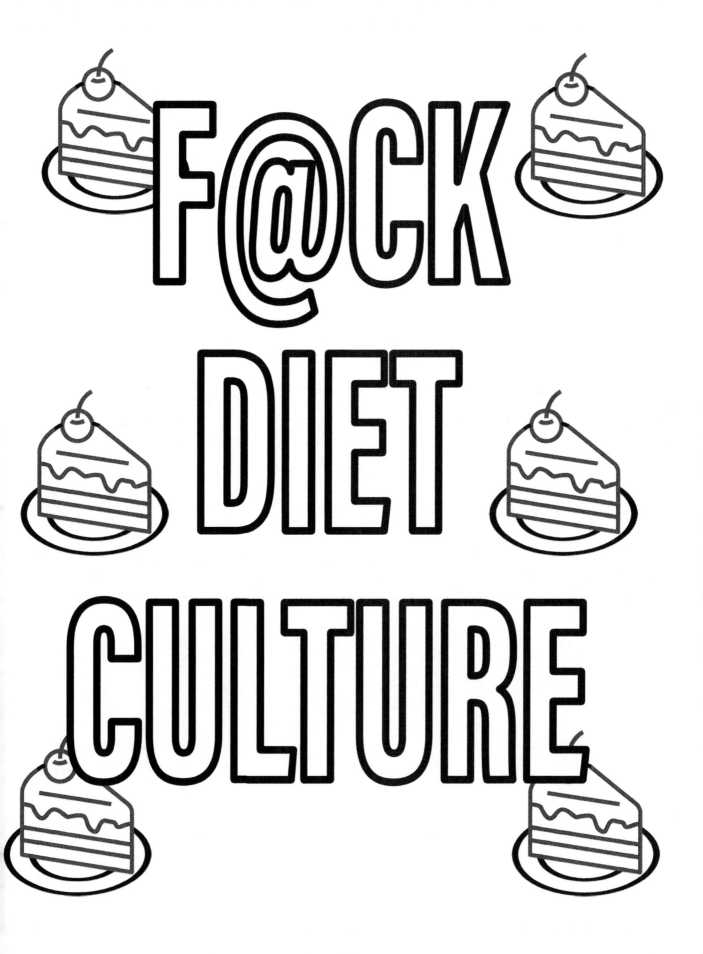

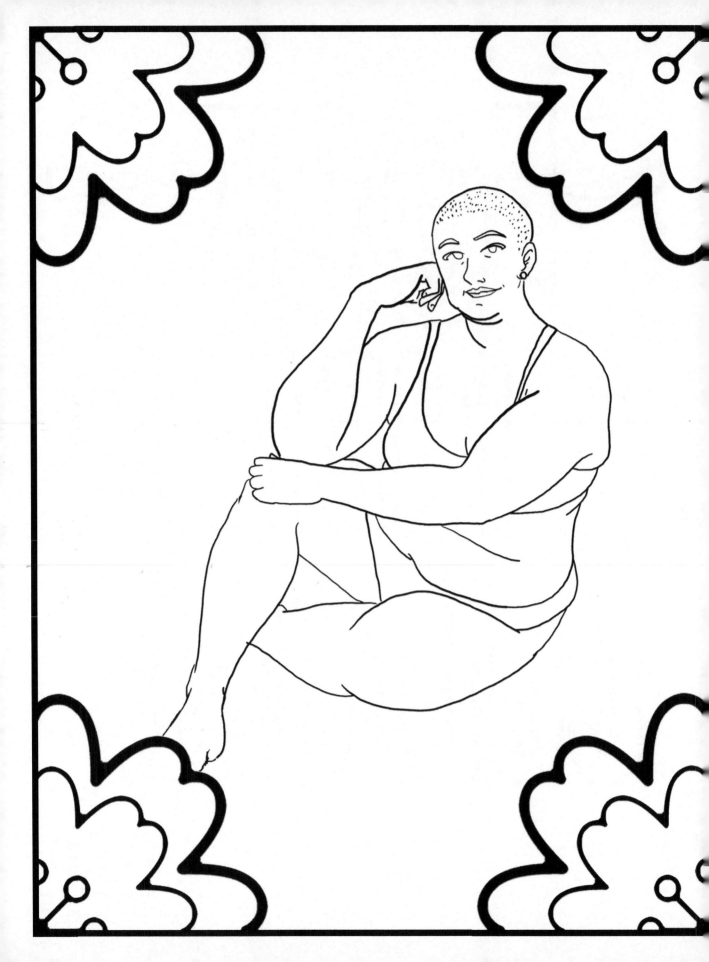

Dear Body,

Write a letter to your body, thank it for all the things it does for you. Compliment what you love about you!

_____

_____

_____

_____

_____

_____

_____

_____

_____

_____

_____

_____

_____

_____

_____

_____

_____

_____

_____

_____

_____

_____

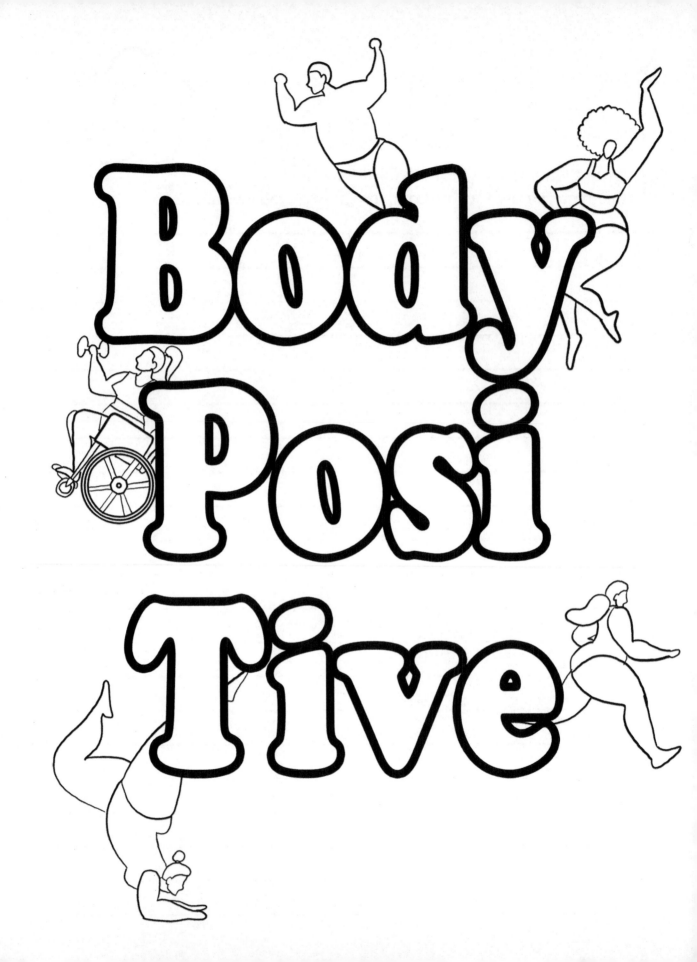